CANCER: My Gift of Self-Actualization!

CANCER: My Gift of Self-Actualization!

✦

How I Converted My Cancer Diagnosis from a Tragedy to a Gift

Rose Marie Duhon-Sells
Contributions by: Glendolyn Duhon-Jeanlouis, Ph.D.

iUniverse, Inc.
New York Lincoln Shanghai

CANCER: My Gift of Self-Actualization!
How I Converted My Cancer Diagnosis from a Tragedy to a Gift

iUniverse books may be ordered through booksellers or by contacting:

iUniverse
2021 Pine Lake Road, Suite 100
Lincoln, NE 68512
www.iuniverse.com
1-800-Authors (1-800-288-4677)

ISBN: 978-0-595-43090-1 (pbk)
ISBN: 978-0-595-87431-6 (ebk)

Printed in the United States of America

For my mother, Alice Duplichain, for her continuous persistence that I did not have any cancer. She remained in denial until her death because the truth was too hard for her to accept. To my husband, Halloway Charles Sells, who supported, nurtured and counseled me through the entire process of the diagnosis, chemotherapy and radiation. He constantly validated my strength and beauty and his key words were, "The most beautiful thing about you is your mind and your heart and the body doesn't even matter." May the souls of both of them rest in peace and their spirits share the glory of this book with me.

Contents

ACKNOWLEDGEMENT

Special thanks also goes out to my four children, Alice Duhon McCullun, Ph.D.; Gwendolyn Mary Duhon, Ph.D.; Glendolyn Mary Jeanlouis, Ph.D. and Patrick Cafrey Duhon, Jr. and seven grandchildren, Donavan, Charles, Grace, Whitney, Brittney, Jordan and Allison who kept my heart smiling and my mind focused on living. I want to express sincere gratitude to the best, most intelligent and supportive administrative assistant, Sally Novatney, who encouraged me to complete this thirteen year old document and pulled it together for me.

FOREWORD

Cancer is every human being's worst nightmare. The sound of the voice that says: "I hate to tell you this, but the test shows that the tumor is cancerous" is never forgotten by the person who is listening to that diagnosis. I was blessed with the ability to turn the devastating message into a "gift of self-actualization" which was nothing more than an effective coping skill for me. It forced me to develop the perception that the experience of having cancer could only make the rest of my life better. The process of doing this includes treasuring all of God's gifts on a daily basis, from the ability to wake up in the morning feeling fine, to inhaling fresh clean air and observing the flowers, trees and grass and recognizing the inspiring, uplifting daily happiness that these provide.

This booklet was written on the premise that any individual diagnosed with any form of cancer may read this and gain a glimmer of hope and attain the strength and inspiration to fight this disease with all their will, desire and commitment. It is amazing when a person is struggling with thoughts of immortality based on the fact that so many people are dying daily from cancer what one word or a positive message from a survivor can do in terms of helping one to see the light at the end of this tunnel. The words in this booklet were written over a 13 year span. There were days when the brightest thing in my day was the opportunity to write my story hoping that it would help someone else to have the courage to write and create their own story.

The message in this booklet isn't meant for individuals of any specific religion, culture, sex, race or creed. Cancer is a disease that does not discriminate. When cancer infiltrates the human body it interferes with the body, soul and the spirit; therefore, if the words in this booklet will help one person to realize that the diagnosis of cancer means to them whatever they decide. Based on the information in this document it is obvious that I decided to turn it into my gift of self-actualization to make my life better, brighter and more meaningful.

INTRODUCTION

Cancer, My Gift of Self-Actualization, is a chronicle of how the diagnosis of cancer was converted into a gift rather than a tragedy. The diagnosis of cancer caused me to reevaluate the meaning of my "life" and "living". The choices I was making about what was important, worth my time, energy and thinking, were sincerely restructured. February, 2004, my 39 year old daughter was diagnosed with level one Breast Cancer. I felt blessed to be able to help her recognize the Gift without wasting valuable time moaning and groaning about "Why me?"

The worst news for any woman is the news of breast cancer. The myth by which we are all affected is that African American women are some of the sexiest women on the globe. Therefore, the breast is a major part of the whole body as we psychologically view ourselves and our sexuality. I think denial is one of the reasons that the death rate for African American women from breast cancer is higher than that of women of other races. We refuse to accept it, so we do not get help. Consequently, we must seek information through research, reading self-help books, listening to courageous, beautiful African Americans who have survived breast cancer and maintained loving, caring, and meaningful relationships with their mates. We need to view our greatness as much more than only our physical appearance and focus on the whole person inside and out. This book has information on strategies appropriate for easing the physical, emotional, and mental pain and fear associated with the first reaction to the cancer diagnosis.

When I was diagnosed, the truth, logic, or the fact of cancer did not come into play for a few months. I, too, was trapped in the myth. The major objective of this book is to motivate, stimulate, and encourage you who are diagnosed with any type of cancer to take charge of your lives and to develop a plan of action to fight for your lives, no matter what it takes. The first step is to talk to survivors, people in holistic medicine and strengthen your faith by believing in yourself and your ability to win this fight.

I believe that our feelings are often controlled by our thinking, and our emotional state is often determined by what we allow ourselves to focus on for periods of time. If you believe "God will turn this diagnosis to good" it will happen. You will experience a level of strength you have and knew you had within you. You will not allow your mind to think about anything other than ways to conquer this cancer. Therefore, I have developed techniques that work for me to ensure that my thinking is forever positive, creative and productive. I realize that there is always a bright side to any given situation. If I spend time thinking about how bad this is and planning my death I will always be down and depressed and that type of thinking will take my strength and energy. The other side is that if I view cancer as a gift, which I have to learn how to conquer, my husband and I will live together for many healthy and happy years. When I wake up in the morning the first thought is what new things I will learn about alternative treatments so that I may improve the quality of my life and that of others. Always share anything you know and learn about treatments with everyone you meet.

This book offers many strategies for selecting and changing your state of mind. The key is to believe that God is in charge of all things on earth, and we are capable of being in control of our minds and bodies. It is most important to believe in the power of God and in your ability to implement the power of prayer as the major source of health and ability to conquer this cancer which is only a disease. I am convinced that there are many simple things we can do to alleviate minor pain associated with cancer, such as headaches or muscles pains, etc. Many of those aches are not related to cancer; they are all in the mind.

I realize that some people may think that I pray regularly and still I encountered cancer. They may use that as an excuse to sit around feeling sorry for themselves and complaining, which is only negative energy that makes matters worst by weakening your ability to progress with your healing and quest to conquer.

The power of prayer must be realized by each one of us in our own unique way. I spend much of my time in prayer when I am alone in my car, waiting in line at a department store, or sitting at home alone. My gift of self-actualization helped me to create a new, stronger, more giving and successful person. I relate everything small and large as being a result of my prayer and my faith which allows me to accept life as it is so I can focus on the positive. This focus on the power of prayer enhances my positive thinking and improves the quality of my life. I attempt to change only those things in my scope of control and move forward with those so that my life is fulfilled and I get the most joy and blessing possible in each day that I am on this earth. This is one of the gifts of my "self actualization" that I have received as a result of breast cancer.

Remedies:

In the early years, people did not have access to modern medical treatments and home remedies. For me the remedies with the medical treatments worked. I researched everything possible. I discovered there are very effective home remedies which will make a difference in the way you feel. One's quality of life is very important when you are dealing with cancer-related illnesses, as well as those only in your mind. This does not mean that you ignore the traditional cancer treatment but it does help if you really believe in it as an effective treatment. My doctor told me if you think something will help you, try it. The key is that you take charge of your health and that gives you a sense of empowerment, you feel like you have some control in your life. You may consider all forms of treatment—alternative cancer treatment is partly responsible for my life today.

I was misdiagnosed in 1992-1993. The cancer was at "level 3" with two "noggles" in my left breast. I had surgery. In 1996, my doctor found a "noggle" in my right breast. By that time I had learned about a black and yellow salve. This remedy drew out the tumor and surgery was not necessary. The medical community did not acknowledge this remedy, nonetheless, no one could tell me where the "noggle" went; it was no longer there. Some people laugh or put this type of treatment down; however, all I want is to live, and I will use anything that works and does not harm.

Research has shown that cancer survivors who pray and/or meditate, use acupuncture, positive visualization and exercise daily yoga tend to have longer lives. This book will have a chapter totally focused on bible verses, short prays and affirmatives appropriate for meditation.

There is information focused on home remedies and many household items that help in easing simple pains such as colds or flu and lack of energy due to cancer survivors' weak immune system. There are many simple mind and body exercises that will provide immediate relief: a song, a walk, pictures of loved ones, etc.

It is important for cancer survivors to follow the directions of their medical doctor. Keep all of your appointments and do not take any supplements for 2 hours after taking any medication. This is a brief description of my daily routine of supplements:

1. I take Genesis by Symmetry[1] twice a day

   • It strengthens my immune system and supports healthy cell regeneration

2. Ultra Vitality by Symmetry once a day

   • A nutritional multi-vitamin and mineral drink with aloe

3. I visit the acupuncturist every six months

---

1. I buy this from Mrs. Frankie Cade—(713) 734-0374

4. I soak cactus leaves (the prickly ones) in my daily drinking water

5. I take Aloe Vera juice with a clove of chopped up garlic every night (the garlic before the juice)

6. I drink green tea daily

7. I take a multitude of vitamins: such as C, E, Q10 and Centrum

1

HISTORICAL OVERVIEW OF MY LIFE

My life began as the youngest of four daughters on a farm in Opelousas, Louisiana, in February, 1941. My grandparents were slaves in "Plaque Point" (not on the map) and my parents were hardworking, wonderful people who did not have the opportunity to get an education. Nevertheless they were determined that their children would be educated. I have three older sisters and two of us have Doctorate degrees and three of my children have PhD's. The open air environment was a gift I have always treasured and even more now that I have had the experience of having cancer and becoming a cancer survivor. I realize how fortunate it was to be born into a loving, caring, and nurturing family. My parents always found a way to let us know they believed in each one of us and they expected great things of us because we were "Duplichains" growing up. I was not certain what that meant but it always made me feel special and capable of conquering any challenge that confronted me. Consequently, that strength helped me in my battle with breast cancer.

My parents were farmers with limited resources, but we did not view ourselves as being poor. We were always well-dressed, clean and focused how we may help others. My mother was the most creative person of her time. She would collect floral flour sacks and design the most beautiful outfits for us to wear, and she could make a simple meal into a delicacy. The atmosphere was one of gratitude and appreciation, not of complaining or focusing on what we did not have. She told stories that always ended with a solid lesson in positive discipline and faith in God.

The life of the youngest was always different than that of the older siblings. The older sisters viewed the baby as the recipient of all the attention and having life so easy. However, they felt a sense of responsibility for me also. My parents expected them to provide me with some special attention even though physically

I was larger than my sister who was a little older. Still I had the label of the "the baby" of the family.

My father, Oneil Duplichain, 6'5" tall, was a handsome, kind, loving, patient man, and very knowledgeable. He never got angry or upset about anything or with anyone. I knew he was the best daddy in the world. Unfortunately, in August of 1947, he had a massive stroke and three days later he passed away. Even though he was in much pain he never complained. His only concern was for my mother and the four of us; he lived for his family. My father was an example of parenting with love and laughter. He would address misbehavior with a funny story that always had a plot focused on a lesson reflecting the disadvantages of misbehavior and how the behavior of each one of us impacted the lives of the total Duplichain family. He told us about family members who had achieved against major odds, always ending the story by saying "and you will be successful as Duplichain women." I now reflect on those days with the academic knowledge I have received as an educator that my father was preparing us for life. Throughout my life when the going gets tough, I think "what would my father do about this."

Now, when I reflect on my father's life, I understand where I inherited my resistance to pain and my determination not to complain ("Why me?") about what I don't have or what is wrong. He taught me early, life is what you think it is, so it is good. At the time of my father's death, I was six years old, and I was told that I was in the process of trying to find solutions to our family problems by asking questions that would help my mother.

We lived on a farm where the beauty of nature is always present with clean air, beautiful greenery, and flowers in bloom year round. I was blessed to be born healthy and develop happy as a child. August was the middle of the harvesting season, mother said, and I was asking any relatives to come to live with us to help my Mama harvest the crops and make my Mama happy again. Unfortunately, after my father's death we could no longer live on that farm; at that time single women were not allowed to stay on the farm without a man to lead the family.

My father was only 42 years of age when he died leaving my mother to be head of household at age 38, with four children all under the age of seventeen. Although she was very strong, smart, and hard working, this was a very difficult role for her because she was not highly educated. (Mother—Alice Greene Duplichain—was one of fourteen children. My grandfather decided that because they lived ten miles from the nearest school for "colored children" his daughters were going to stay home and the boys would go to school and learn how to read and write so that when they were men they could best provide for their families. The thinking then was that the girls would always have husbands to take care of them.)

Nevertheless, my mother was the best parent, counselor, teacher, and provider that I have ever known. She had a way of addressing problematic issues through telling stories every night as we sat near the fireplace and these would always have a real life plot that focused on a life skill. When she sensed a problem developing around one of us or that would affect the family structure, she would gather the family around the oldtime clay fireplace and put sweet potatoes wrapped in foil at the edge of the flames and we would talk for hours. The discussion always included a Bible verse or a song and what life would be like when we completed our education and became professional women.

She was 94 years old and still talked about how hard it was to accept my father's death. It caused my mother to have to work two and three low-paying jobs to ensure that we always had enough to eat and that we were appropriately dressed for school and especially for church. She spent all of her time with us, and I did not realize how lonely she must have been without a mate. She decided soon after my father's death that she would not remarry because she did not want to take the risk of exposing her girls (the four of us) to a strange man who might look at us, or even touch us, inappropriately. At that time, many of her family and friends thought that she was foolish and would change her mind, but 65 years later she kept to the promise. However, the current media stories of the sexual misbehavior of many stepfathers have caused me to think that my mother had reason to be cautious. Reflecting on the past, I have followed in her footsteps; when my first husband died, I did not remarry until all of my children were out of school and themselves married.

I learned at an early age that life is not perfect. My parents prepared me for that reality. There will be hard times, they said, but with strong faith in the Lord Jesus Christ, believing in yourself, getting all the education available, treating everyone you meet with dignity and respect you will achieve anything you want as long as mistakes are viewed as learning opportunities. Know that you are as good as anyone else and do not allow anyone to cause you to think otherwise.

Our family attended church every Sunday and other religious holy days during the week. No one in my family was allowed to curse or fight in the presence of my mother. She hated any kind of sibling conflict. She believed all problems could be solved by talking about them in a positive way. Everyday, we started with a family prayer and ended the day with family prayer at night. The family always worshipped together on holidays, and the major events of our families were planned around church activities. Therefore, I grew up on faith and faith helped me to reverse the tragedy of cancer from a destroyer to a gift of life. When life gets tough, my faith always provides me with the comfort of knowing I have the power of God on my side, waiting for me to ask and immediately receive the needed help to move from negative to positive. God knows what we need. We do not always get what we ask for, because some of the things we may ask for in God's eyes may not be the best thing for us at that time. God knows the future, we do not. All we have is the strength and knowledge of the present.

I started school at four years old because my mother worked in the cafeteria and had no one to take care of me during the day. So I went with my sisters and participated in all the activities. I attended Biagas Elementary, a Louisiana rural elementary school, which had very few academic resources. We had to walk three miles each way and sometimes we were teased and ridiculed by other children.

But our teachers had a way of making us feel special, that we were beautiful and smart and ensuring us that we could do anything if we were willing to work hard and listen carefully to the instructors. All students experienced success daily. We were loved and appreciated. Even if it were only reading one sentence correctly, the teachers focused on enhancing the student's self-esteem by acknowledging their strength and that was not a buzz word then. They created special events weekly which included participation of the family, so that each student had a unique task to perform. These activities made the student think and feel that no one else in the world could accomplish these tasks more effectively than, or as well as, they could.

My elementary school years were most fulfilled in the eighth grade. Toward the end of the year, my mother decided to move to a small town (Lawtell, Louisiana). I had to attend high school in Opelousas, Louisiana, which was a large city in comparison to Plaque Point where I grew up and attended elementary school. I was a star in my elementary school (Biagas Elementary). Unfortunately, when I transferred to J. S. Clark High School in Opelousas, I felt unaccepted, different, and was a stranger. I felt that I did not "fit in" in the city or in the school culture of the student population. The other students were basically from the inner city and teased us about being "country." Consequently, we were coming from a culture filled with all the resources in terms of harvested foods and a strong value system with high morals. Most of them had experienced the pains of poverty, and we were the target of their anger and limitation. Unfortunately, at that time I did not understand and it hurt not to belong. The classes were large and the teachers were cold and distant. The students were basically from local feeder elementary schools in the area, so they all seemed to know each other, and I was not a part of the inner circle.

After a few years, I dropped out of high school in the eleventh grade, got married, and ten years later, I had given birth to five lovely children, three girls and two boys, all of whom are well grounded, successful and carrying the legacy of my strong early experiences. I lost my oldest son in a tragic accident in 1962, which was devastating and is still current in my mind, as though it occurred yesterday. I think of him almost daily. My faith in God pulled me through that experience, and I learned to live with his memories. I really believe that my baby is in Heaven with God and his spirit watches over me and my family. I often pray asking him to pray for us, for he is closer to God in His kingdom than we are. I believe that he has guided me to recognize my experience with the cancer as a gift of actualization—one that helps me to enjoy life in depth and helps me to acknowledge what is important for me to get the most out of life. The key is that I believe God has a special task for me to perform and that is to help others accept the news of cancer as a message to improve the quality of their lives.

The year my youngest entered pre-school, I soon realized that I suffered from the "empty nest" syndrome. I no longer felt needed or worthwhile. My major job responsibility was over. I had no real reason to stay home all day and when my husband (who had two jobs) came home, I had nothing of significance to share about my day. There were limited options for employment without an earned high school diploma, and generally, the respect for common knowledge, did not exist; even though there are smart people who have never attended formal school. The society we live in is a degree-certified culture. Even though a person is knowledgeable, he must be validated with a degree to be respected and accepted. Actually, if a person does not have a high school diploma, some view him/her as not real thinkers in this society. I disagree with that theory, but we must live in the real world. Therefore, I decided to inquire about attending adult education. Fortunately, I went to the local school to find one of my former elementary school teachers, Mrs. Thelma Allen, in charge of the adult education program. She built me up immediately by saying, "Girl, you have a good head on your shoulders, you are very smart, and you were one of my best students. Why did you drop out of school?" I could not start telling her the real reason because I did not understand until I later began studying the cognitive development of the young mind.

How could I find the words to tell Mrs. Allen the real reason for dropping out of school? At that time I had no answer for the question. When I later studied brain-based learning, I recognized that because I was emotionally paralyzed, my brain had shut down, and I could no long learn in that J. S. Clark High School environment. Sadly, today many smart students are leaving school for the same reason and they, too, do not know why.

My old teacher immediately helped me to regain the confidence I had experienced in the process of growing up in Plaque Point at Biagas Elementary School. She gave me the important missing elements to open my brain and start it functioning at its normal level once again.

I took a series of placement examinations to determine which classes I should be placed in to complete my high school studies and I scored two years of college. I immediately received my General Equivalency Diploma (GED). A few months later, I enrolled in college and four years later I received a Bachelor of Arts Degree at the University of Southwestern Louisiana. USL was a predominately white school and I experienced racism, but it did not impact my brain as much as the isolation did because I was an adult who had a mission to succeed.

Returning to school as an adult with four children and a husband was very challenging, but I was determined and committed to succeed. I received a scholarship which helped with tuition. However, in the Sixties, attending a recently integrated university was an experience I shall never forget. The rejection, disrespect, and mean spirited treatment which I endured have served to help me to become a stronger person, and I realized this world does not encourage a person of color to move ahead; that is God's task. I soon realized that I was strong enough to succeed under those conditions, and I knew that I was capable of earning other degrees in any institutional environment. I turned the negative to the positive and focused on the bottom line—to graduate as soon as I could. I viewed racism as a problem God would handle for me.

I taught elementary school for seven years and during that time, I also attended Southern University, where I received a master's degree in Guidance and Counseling. I later specialized in Administration and Supervision. My accomplishments were with the assistance, encouragement, and support of my husband, Patrick Cafrey Duhon, Sr., who truly believed in me. He was a real provider for the family. He was kind, loving, and very knowledgeable. He knew how to manage money better than the average CPA. Because of him I knew I had the ability to earn my degree and deal with any obstacle in my path without falling under pressures.

In 1978, my husband of twenty years died, leaving me with four children aged 16, 13, 13, and 11. I was lost because he was the leader of the family, my lover, advisor, friend, and role model. I learned so much from him; he was everything to me. He was a great father, and the children loved and respected him so that he never had to lift his voice with them. When he walked in, they knew their behavior had to change or the chores had to be completed because he did not accept any excuses. Nevertheless, the positive developmental foundation my mother had created and instilled in me again provided the strength needed to help me to snap back to reality to the responsibility of caring, providing, and guiding through life those four children who were now all mine and by the Grace of God, I knew we would survive. I prayed and received God's guidance to create a new and different life for us in this world without him, but with his spirit in our hearts and a life provided greater challenges and rewards.

I spent time grieving and reflecting on my deceased husband's philosophy, which was to teach our children that with love and understanding they would develop into caring, independent adults. He believed that if you use your money wisely and always save something every payday, even if it is only ten ($10) dollars, you would never be in a real financial bind. He was so right; to this day I remind my children of their father's great budgeting skills and hope they will develop them and become financially independent adults. He also believed that no matter what happens in life, if you look forward and focus on God's Power, there will be a brighter day. He and my mother had a lot in common in that both were great budgeters and both believed in the power of God to solve all problems big and small. Now that both are gone, I am determined to carry the legacy to the family and the next level.

I realized that one complemented the other, and it was as though my twenty years of marriage was the opportunity to implement the life skills my mother taught me in a loving and supporting partnership with the man I loved. I was blessed by God to have gotten married at sixteen to a young man of eighteen, and we grew up together in God's will, sharing the good and the bad times for twenty beautiful years. Our relationship was deeper than that of any husband and wife because we shared our faith. The year my husband passed away, circumstances caused me to revamp my whole life. I experienced the feeling of having the world on my shoulders. I was responsible for the survival and well-being of my family—four children—at their most critical ages. As teenagers, children need so much love, support and attention. The hard part is that they resist what they need most and as parents we must fight them to help them.

I was in contact with my major professor from my master's degree in Guidance and Counseling, Dr. Laura Beth Hicks, from Southern University. Dr. Hicks is a genius and committed to helping students attain their highest life goals; she was my mentor. She suggested that I enroll in a doctoral program and study for a Ph.D. degree. After many conversations, much encouragement and support, I decided to apply to Kansas State University and was accepted. I took my four children on a month's vacation to Manhattan, Kansas, to help the family to decide if they wanted to live there for two years. After two weeks, the family decided that we would move to Kansas so I could study at Kansas State University to earn my Ph.D. in Education. At that time, I became driven as a mother to ensure that I would create appropriate life experiences for my children that provided them with many options in life so that they could be educated, independent, comfortable, and major contributions to society. Life as a single parent was demanding. I had to make a major life decision, which was to remain in the comfort of my extended family where I was supported, loved and assisted with my children or branch out into an unfamiliar world with my four teenage children to create a new life with a greater opportunities for them to imitate and participate in the mainstreams of life. I spent time praying for guidance, and God, as always, guided us all the way. There were bumps in the road, but we endured.

The day we were moving to Kansas, my furniture was on the U-Haul truck, the phone rang; it was the Dean of the College of Education at Kansas State calling to inform me that the scholarship which was promised to me was not funded; the University had no money to help me with tuition, so do not come to Kansas. I told him that I had rented my house, sold my husband's car and most of my things; therefore, I was coming to Kansas and I was going to wait on the money. Most importantly, I had promised my children that we were moving. He tried to discourage me, but to no avail. We arrived in Manhattan, Kansas, on a Saturday and I was in the Dean's office every weekday for the next two weeks. On the Monday of the third week, I started the routine again. Fortunately, I burned the Dean out; he told his secretary to give me anything I wanted and added that with that determination, it was well deserved. He said in the history of his administration he had never experienced a person (a mother) with that level of determination.

I took advantage of this opportunity and enrolled for twenty college credit hours in the graduate school that first semester as well, sewed for my children, helped them with their school work and worked often as a substitute teacher in the local public school. This was to ensure that my children's needs were met. I had one daughter in college at Southern University at that time. I would stay up nights until 2:00 a.m. to make new wardrobes for her to take with her to college each season. Money was limited. We worked together, talked about our needs, and we always had enough of everything, food, clothes, etc. My family in Louisiana supported and encouraged us every step of the way as did many great people we met along the way. With my strong faith in God, I did earn my degree (December, 1978) and provided for my children through their challenging teen years. The best life experience ever is that three of my four children now have earned Ph.D. degrees.

This is the point when I lost sight of "me" as a person with needs and only focused on being a good provider, parent, and head of my family. In Kansas we attended Church services every Sunday, and I attended Mass as often as possible. I was my children's role model. They learned skills in how to deal with life issues that are beyond one's control. Therefore, when I was diagnosed with breast cancer, they felt comfortable that I would be fine. I realized that this was an impossible task that was possible only through the power of God's answers to my prayers. I was so committed to my children, focused on helping them to fulfill their life dreams and to reach the goals which my husband and myself had set for them. I was worried that they would miss some of life's opportunities because they had lost their father. To this day I get upset when I hear people use the fact that growing up in a single parent family did not give them the necessary commitment, determination, or confidence in themselves to strive for success. My life is an example of meeting the needs of children by giving them love, support and attention.

I immersed myself in my work, and my health and well-being became secondary. I rationalized away any symptoms I had and procrastinated in making doctor's appointments. Therefore, I did not have the balance in my life that ensures a healthy, fulfilled life that addresses self needs as well as other responsibilities. At that time I believed that the only way for my children to succeed was for me to show them it could be done against the odds.

The term "workaholic" is not a joke; it is an illness, one that may lead to more serious illness like cancer. Consequently, when you enjoy giving of yourself, make sure that you have the best mind, body and spirit to share. I often think that my cancer diagnosis was God's way of telling me that I had far exceeded the expectations of my family, even for a parent. The key to success is to recognize your blessings daily and work to be a blessing to others.

I had a full-time position as a professor, where I was teaching three to four college-level graduate and undergraduate courses. I was conducting research on several topics such as multicultural education, child abuse and neglect, effective parenting skills, and effective teaching strategies for teachers of young children. I published my first article in 1980 on "Child Abuse" and my first book in 1985 entitled *Teaching Young Children to Love Learning with TYCME*, which is the acronym for Teaching Young Children About Multicultural Education. I enjoyed learning so much about a topic that reflected my thinking, about how everyone needs to be accepted, respected and embraced as valuable human beings that I got very excited about building my foundation and extending areas for me. I was the first person in the history of my family (maternal and paternal) to become an author of an academic book. I was invited to speak at conferences across the globe, i.e., Paris, France; Australia, South Africa, Asia, and Italy. I felt as though I had to take advantage of everything offered to me to best represent my grandparents, who were slaves.

In spite of their experience of a life that is unbelievable to me, through their love, teachings and support they created a life legacy for me that helps me to dream and aspire to a life of giving, caring and a determination to change and improve the quality of life for others.

Cancer, My Gift of Self-Actualization, is a story which, I think, will de-mystify the fear or the belief that cancer attacks only certain kinds of people. The fear, when a person is diagnosed with cancer, is that life will change for the worse. The fear that after the cancer is diagnosed, you will become limited in your creative thinking or ability to have new innovative ideas that will create positive changes in this world. Another myth is that if people know you are a cancer survivor, your job options will be limited, you will be viewed as weak and a bad risk or not strong enough to endure or roll with the flow of the daily duties. This will only happen if a cancer survivor uses the "cancer" as a tool to get pity or special treatment from other people including employers. This behavior will hurt the person more than the cancer will. It is not helpful.

2

THE CRITICAL NEWS

In 1993, I was living in Baton Rouge, Louisiana. One Tuesday morning when I woke-up I felt a strong pain in my right breast and my husband begged me, "Please go to the doctor today, something is wrong with you." I said, "Not today, honey, I am too busy." But later that morning I decided I'd better see the doctor, to get my husband off my time. This was the beginning of the process of living with the daily commitment, determination and faith to conquer my cancer.

When I arrived at the doctor's office, I told the doctor that my schedule was full for the next four months and I could not make an appointment with her until July. I felt that I was at the peak of my career and the world would stop without my presence. I was the Founder and First President of a major national organization, the National Association for Multicultural Education, which was blossoming into the largest education organization in this country. Also I had been recently elected National President of the oldest and most prestigious national organization for educators, the Association of Teacher Educators (ATE), the first African American to serve in that position in their 77-year history. I had entered my third year of a second marriage to a wonderful man who shared my faith, interest, and commitment to improving our quality of life for everyone who needed us. All four of my children had attended college. Three were college grad-uates, all were married with stable jobs and happy families. Two of my children were in graduate school working on doctoral degrees. I had reached the highest academic level of recognition; I was nationally acknowledged as a scholar, leader and I was respected and admired by my peers across the globe. I had exceeded my highest academic goals. I had gone from a high school dropout, to an honor roll student throughout four years of college, to a college professor, author, national lecturer and scholar in the field of Education. Many people were amazed at my determination and accomplishments as the granddaughter of slaves. They did not know that some of the world's smartest students drop out of school because they do not feel loved, supported or accepted. The school system is not designed to address or fulfill the most important emotional needs of students or when they are not academically challenged by the teachers or school personnel. This does not say that I wasn't gifted, but I know that I was not motivated and very bored. My outlet was marriage. I thank God for intervening and providing me with a great mate. I was one of those students hurt by schooling and no one—teacher, principal or anyone else—noticed. Unfortunately, so many other dropouts do not land on their feet, with a second chance as I did.

I was in my fourth year as the Dean of the College of Education at Southern University, Baton Rouge. Many of the projects I had implemented were successful. My children were grown, married, and successful. My family was growing with six grandchildren. Everyone was healthy, happy, and prosperous; I felt that life was as close to perfect as I wanted it to be with little or no worries. I was working harder than ever before; I rationalized that I needed to help everyone in need of my services because I had the knowledge, energy, and compassion necessary to make life better for all. The College of Education was experiencing some major problems such as in-fighting among faculty and I felt I was improving that climate.

My breast had been sensitive for a few weeks, but I was hesitant about going to the doctor because I did not have the time, I was too busy. I felt confident that it was only something minor and it was going to be all right because only eleven months earlier I had gone for a mammogram and was told "everything is fine, see you in a year." (Unfortunately, the X-ray had been misread.) Nevertheless, my husband asked me to go to my gynecologist that day so that he could have peace of mind. He was very concerned because he felt that what I was experiencing was not normal. I first thought that he was just a worrier, but because I loved him I would go to let the doctor tell me again that I was fine. I had three appointments that morning, one of which was a one hour interview on the radio about multicultural education issues, which was a very controversial topic all over the country and more so in Louisiana. My stress level has always been high even though I thought positive stress was acceptable and did not negatively affect the body. I was wrong. Too much of any kind of stress is bad for our physical, emotional, and mental stability. The doctor examined me at a clinic in Baton Rouge. After the mammogram, the doctor said that it was just scar tissue from giving birth to five children. I thought that that did not make sense because my youngest child was twenty-eight (28) years old. I tried not to entertain that thought because this was an HMO; they did not care about their patients. I insisted on having a mammogram immediately. The technician seemed very concerned. She repeated the procedure at least three times. The next day, the doctor tracked me down to return for biopsies. I immediately dropped the HMO and made an appointment with Dr. Laura Cassidy. I was told she was the best cancer specialist in Baton Rouge. The results of the exam showed that there was a lump and I needed to be checked by a cancer specialist. The nurse asked me when I could schedule an appointment because surgery had to be performed to remove the lump. I looked in my appointment book and saw that I was booked for the next four months. I guess you can say that I had become a "work alcoholic."

By February 12, 1993, three days had past since the biopsies and I was anxious about the results of the test. My daughter was getting married at six o'clock that evening in Houston, Texas. It was about 2 o'clock in the afternoon when I decided to phone Dr. Cassidy. She did not have to tell me the diagnosis; I heard it in her voice. She is the most caring, compassionate, and professional person I have ever met. She comforted me without being patronizing or sympathetic. She treated me as a fellow professional. I asked her how long I had to live. She answered, "Well you may live into your seventies depending on the type and stage of the cancer." I did not know how to end the conversation so she told me to call her when I got home. I felt a sense of emptiness, loneliness and sadness all at once. I started missing my family and friends immediately. I had no knowledge of how to deal with this news. I had no one in my family who had gone through this experience. My first thought was "I am going to die and all that I have done is to work long hours fighting trivial battles with many insignificant people who did not care whether I lived or died". I soon realized that what I was doing was not important to anyone. Then I stopped thinking about death and started to pray, asking God to help me to accept the diagnosis. The next thought I had was, "What will I do about this illness?" I started questioning, "How will I fight this?"

Those thoughts helped me to feel stronger, more positive, and generated some hope. I became empowered. The total helplessness started to subside ever so slightly. My immediate reaction was to think about my daughter's special day, her wedding. I could not share this news with anyone until after the wedding event. I felt they would not be able to keep their emotions in control throughout the wedding. I am blessed to have a sister, Mary Mandel, with whom I could share the news immediately. We are very close and, because of her strong will, I felt she would be the one for me to tell. I gave her a call and told her the results of the examination. We both cried. In my heart, I knew that everything would be fine. Because of my sister's caring personality, she immediately offered to assume some of my role as mother of the bride. This was great because she has such a good relationship with my daughters. My daughter did not even notice that my sister was taking charge of the task which I would normally perform. She made it possible that no one even noticed I was sad and upset. I pretended all was well.

The wedding was beautiful and everyone had a good time. It was hard at times for me to totally concentrate on the wedding. But I gave it my best shot and pretended that everything was just great. I knew in the back of my mind that I had to tell the family first thing Sunday morning. I told some of my children that night. We all gathered around the table in the kitchen where I proceeded to tell the children about the test results. I assured them that everything was going to be all right. Internally, I was frightened, unsure, and lost as to how I was going to be able to control this thing called cancer. To me this word meant death.

I am writing this book so that others will be assured that the news of cancer will not be as devastating for them as it was for me. In 2004, when my daughter was diagnosed, I helped her to accept it and start the healing process.

3

THE HEALING POWER OF GOD

This chapter must start with my favorite Bible verses to read daily as a strong source of uplifting strength. Reading the following verses help to start a wonderful day with the ability to acknowledge the many blessings bestowed on each of us daily:

LUKE 21:1-28
PSALM1:1-6
PSALM 23:1-6
PSALM 69:1-14
PSALM 90:1-91:16

I have always found strength in my faith in God, because, I grew up in the church. However, when I learned that I had cancer, my faith was tested. Initially, the first few days I would pray and cry, trying to identify a reason, or something I had done to deserve this horrible disease at the peak of my life. I had thought everything was nearly perfect. Soon, I moved from the pit of self-pity and started thanking God for leading me through this experience by loving and protecting me all the way, reassuring me that through it all His presence would always be there with me. I started praying more, talking to God the way I talked to a trusted, kind, and caring friend. I used visual imagery to move my thinking to visualize the Holy Spirit healing my body with the precious blood of Jesus. When I had chemotherapy treatments, I used this method to help my body to accept and respond positively to the treatments without getting really sick with nausea as many of my friends did who were also taking chemotherapy. At that moment, I started seeking to identify the daily miracles which God made in my life. I noticed His hand in everything, the little things as well as the big things. I began to concentrate on the bible's messages and change my belief system to see things from the perspective of faith and not the perspective of science. I became focused on positive thinking about life and living. God helped me to gain strength as He has helped other cancer patients through counseling and praying. I met many young people at the doctor's office and in the community who were devastated about being diagnosed with cancer. They were very afraid of death and dying. This was not easy for me because I was taught that my faith was very secretive and private. We were always reminded that Catholics were very quiet in their praying, and it was inappropriate to openly express your love and gratitude to God for the many gifts provided, such as, strength, comfort, and happiness.

I grew up in the Catholic Church attending mass on Sundays and holy days of obligation. However, I learned the real meaning of the power of God, which we experienced through prayer during the past five years following my cancer diagnosis. I have had the opportunity to think about death, dying, and living. I have reflected on the many miracles which God provides daily which we often take for granted. I have learned to see the power of God's work in every event of my life—the good things and the bad things. A doctor at M. D. Anderson's Cancer Hospital asked me to what did I attribute my survival of cancer, because I had two different kinds—one aggressive and one not so aggressive. I told him that my survival was a result of my strong faith in God. He answered by telling me that many people pray and still they have died. My response was that when I surrendered my life to God's will, I was prepared to accept anything He placed in my path. Unfortunately, many people do not realize that strong faith creates an acceptance for life **and** death. No one will live forever, but strong faith provides a sense of sincerity, calmness, assuredness and comfort in that God is in charge and all is well, in any state of mind.

I felt strange when I first started praying with people openly, and when I would tell others about the miracles which God made on my life, and when I would help them to recognize God's word in their lives. I had to believe and step beyond myself to do God's work. And I had so many people praying *for* me. In the Catholic Church, we believe in lighting blessed candles and propose masses for our special intentions. The candles burn in the church while family and friends pray for you. When I decided to surrender my life, health, and happiness to the power of God, He brought forth so many opportunities for me to learn about alternative treatments for cancer, i.e., vitamins, teas, exercise, and appropriate diet. The process of being involved in this therapeutic process helped me to control the feelings of helplessness and hopelessness. My faith is the cornerstone of my surviving and physical and psychological strength. When my mind would drift to thinking about the negative side of being a cancer survivor, I would quietly focus on the blessing of God's power and the comfort of His support and the strength which He provides when we are in need. It took me several months to perfect this type of mind control. I had to work on it every day. The moment I started to feel down, I would immediately start reciting the gifts of God for that day, such as, clean air, flowers growing in the woods, a loving family, friends, etc. As this list got longer, the negative thoughts would subside and the bad feelings would slowly go away.

The healing power of God works in my life on a daily basis. There are days when my mind and heart will weigh heavy on issues related to cancer. On those days, I often started praying and my mind would drift to negative thoughts, such as, "why me?" or "cancer is deadly." I would immediately go to my Bible and open it randomly to any page and start reading. Within seconds, I would receive an answer to my prayer, which often lifted my spirits to a love so high that I felt like I wanted to sing. I knew that it was God giving me strength. I have several short prayers that were given to me by concerned family members and friends that I read daily to keep my mind off of myself and on the power of God's gifts.

Whether a person is a cancer survivor, a victim of another disease, or in perfect health, life is filled with high-spirited days and low-spirited days. The way I decide to deal with the low-spirited days determines my quality of life on that day. Consequently, the psychological impact of those mood-swing days are determined by how one deals with the challenge and finds an effective strategy that helps him or her to grow from that particular emotional state. My faith in God is the only way that I can pick myself up at the beginning of this journey to survive cancer. I believe in daily affirmations. The one I use daily to keep my sanity is, "I believe in the Healing Power of the Lord Jesus, that I am healed." When I repeat this several times, I always get rejuvenated and I feel a sense of inner comforting that helps me to move on to something positive.

On the days when I am waiting for medical reports on various tests related to assessments of whether or not I have cancer cells or tumors in my body, I include my family and friends to create a chain of prayer. For example, we would decide that everyone would stop whatever they were doing at 11:00 a.m., and spiritually join in a circle of prayer. When my mother was alive, she would go to a Catholic mass service everyday. Also, she had candles burning in the church, always, where she would go to pray to a particular Saint on a daily basis. I met a woman one day who was dying, and she asked me, "Do you think prayer will keep me from dying?" I answered her by reassuring her that we will all die, but prayer will help you to accept death and help you to conceptualize death as a higher level of spirituality, and that dying is not the end of life but the beginning of eternal life on a higher plan. She was a highly educated person who was a Christian, but she had doubts like many people.

I have developed my own state of mind about death and dying. It helps me to accept my life the way it is in this reality. I did not want to get cancer, but I had it, and I needed to develop a positive relationship with this condition in order to enjoy a meaningful quality of life, where I could focus on living, contributing, and enjoying this only life which I have. Learning about the power of God through the power of prayer has changed, improved, and helped me to be happy. Also, my faith has helped me to help others.

The way that prayer works is to call everyone and ask them to pray for my petition between 6:00 a.m. to 7:00 a.m., for the next three to five days. This power miracle strategy of prayer is very effective in many ways. This is not to say that the answer will always be what I want to hear. But the power of God will provide the strength to endure any findings with a strong will and confidence that I, along with the power of God, can positively face and fight anything I encounter on this earth. My faith in God gives me a higher quality of life in spite of being a cancer survivor. It allows me to function with daily responsibilities; it helps me to avoid "pity parties;" it resolves the feeling of fear and provides rationale for my wondering mind that says, "what if?" There were times when I felt totally out of control of certain situations around me, such as, at the doctor's office or when someone makes a mistake and acts as if it is not a big thing. I am thinking it is my life which is a real "big thing" to me. At that moment, I close my eyes and focus on God, My Lord Jesus Christ. I move in that state by repeating over and over again, Jesus, Jesus, Jesus, Jesus. Within minutes, my perception of the situation has changed from negative to positive. This positive thinking immediately helps me to think on a higher level, with the comfort of feeling empowered and the bad feelings of helplessness and hopelessness dissipated. There are several short affirmations which I use daily, such as, I BELIEVE IN THE HEALING POWER OF JESUS CHRIST, THAT MY BODY IS HEALED. When I first learned about the power of using positive affirmations, I felt foolish and I did not want to share with anyone that I believed something so simple would really work to make me feel better.

This affirmation made me feel better and helped me to move beyond the sad negative thinking that was ruining my quality of life. The questions that were repeated over and over in my mind, I could not answer. "Why me?" "When will I die?" "Will I suffer much before dying?" "What will my family, particularly my children, do without me?" and the list went on and on. Now, my trust in God has helped me to put all the questions and concerns in His hands knowing that all will be most effectively taken care of in the best possible way for all involved. Therefore, I have surrendered my life to God's will and I am a happy "breast cancer survivor."

The results were so great in lifting my spirits from a low where I could barely get out of bed, to a high where I felt like singing a happy song; I realized it was my duty to help others by telling them how well this strategy worked for me. The key is that one must really believe in the affirmation statement. We are all victims of a negative society that focuses on the bad and questions the good in everything; therefore, when we convince our minds that it is beneficial to focus on the positive possibilities then the quality of life is enhanced and we enjoy the simple gifts given to us by God daily.

This is very important for many reasons. A researcher writes that high stress levels are related to the development and reoccurrence of cancer-related diseases. Also, anger places a strain on essential body parts, which is bad for one's health. The following strategies have helped to manage my feelings of anger and minimize the negative effect of those emotions on my body. The following may be helpful to others:

1. Is this worth my sincere attention?

2. Can I change the situation in a positive way by discussing the issue with other parties involved?

3. Is it possible that if I listen, I may learn new information that will provide clarity that will solve this problem?

4. How may I turn this into a "win-win situation"?

5. How will I be big enough to say "I am sorry ... I misunderstood"?

I use my faith to control my emotions. The following are copies of some of the daily prayers that contributed to my blessed state of mind. These are copies of prayers that I use every morning.

SERENITY PRAYER

God, grant me the serenity
To accept the things I cannot change,
The courage to change the things I can,
And the wisdom to know the difference.

Living one day at a time;
Enjoying one moment at a time;
Accepting hardship as a pathway to peace;
Taking, as Jesus did,
This sinful world as it is, Not as I would have it;
Trusting that You will make all things right
If I surrender to Your will;
So that I may be reasonably happy in this life
And supremely happy
With You forever in the next.
Amen.
(Franciscan Mission Associates
P. O. Box 598, Mount Vernon, N. Y. 10551-0598)

PRAYERS FOR GOD'S HEALING POWER

When sickness comes, let faith in God's healing power also come. Read again the many stories in the New Testament. Jesus healed the sick. Yield yourself or your loved one into His hands and truly believe.
(Author Unknown)

PRAYER WHEN A LOVED ONE IS ILL

Dear Lord, our loved one (mention the name) is ill. Touch him, I beseech Thee, with the healing grace of Jesus Christ and make him well.

You have our loved ones life and You have the power to renew his life. We put him in Your kindly and loving hands, knowing that no harm can come to him while in Your care, whether on earth or in heaven.

I believe in Thy power to heal the sick. Through faith the tremendous healing force of God the Creator re-creates. I hold our loved one up to Thee and humbly ask that You will lay Your hands upon him and restore him, even as You did to those about whom we read in the Bible.

Jesus Christ is the same yesterday, today and forever and You, Dear Lord, can give new health and strength to our dear one. This we humbly and earnestly request in Thy holy name. Amen.
(Author Unknown)

JESUS, HELP ME!

In every need let me come to Thee with humble trust, saying Jesus, help me! In all my doubts, perplexities, and temptations Jesus help me! In hours of loneliness, weariness and trials Jesus help me! In the failure of my plans and hopes; in disappointments, troubles and sorrows Jesus, help me!

When others fail me, and Thy Grace alone can assist me Jesus, help me! When I throw myself on Thy Tender Love as a Father and Savior Jesus, help me! When my heart is cast down by failure, at seeing no good come from my efforts Jesus, help me! When I feel impatient, and my cross irritates me Jesus, help me! When I am ill, and my head and hands cannot work and I am lonely Jesus, help me!

Always, always, in spite of weakness, falls and shortcomings of every kind Jesus, help me and never forsake me.

(Priests of the Sacred Heart Sacred Heart Monastery)

PRAYER FOR SELF WHEN ILL

Dear Lord, Thou who art the great physician, I turn to Thee in my sickness asking You to help me.

Put Your hand upon me as You did in the long ago and let health and wholeness come into me from Thee.

I put myself under Your care and affirm my faith that even now Your marvelous healing grace is making me well and strong again.

I know that I ask more than I deserve but You never measure out benefits on that basis. You just love us back into health. Do that for me, I earnestly ask, and I will try to serve You more faithfully. This I promise, through Jesus Christ. Amen.

(Author Unknown)

PRAYER FOR MY DOCTOR

Thank You, O Lord, for my doctor.

Give him insight that he may understand and diagnose. Steady his hand and guide him by Thy strong hand. Look over his shoulder, O Lord, and endow him with power to heal in Thy name, through Jesus Christ our Lord. Amen.

(Author Unknown)

NOVENAS 2011
PRAYER TO THE HOLY SPIRIT

You solve all problems and light all roads so that I can obtain my goals. You who give me the divine gift to forgive and forget all evils against me. In all instances of

life, You are with me. I want in this short prayer, to thank You for all things and to confirm once again that I never want to be separated from You, even in spite of material illusions. I wish to be with You in eternal glory. Thank You for Your mercy towards me and mine. **(Say this prayer for 3 days. After 3 days, favors will be granted even if it appears difficult, Publish prayer immediately after favor has been granted. G.A.R.)**
(Author Unknown)

IN TIME OF NEED

Jesus, do not leave me alone in suffering. You know, Lord, how weak I am. I am an abyss of wretchedness, I am nothingness itself; so what will be so strange if You leave me alone and I fall? I am an infant, Lord, so I cannot get along by myself. However, beyond all abandonment I trust, and in spite of my own feeling I trust, and I am being completely transformed into trust—often in spite of what I feel. Do not lessen any of my sufferings, only give me strength to bear them. Do with me as You please, Lord, only give me the grace to be able to love You in every event and circumstance. Lord, do not lessen my cup of bitterness, only give me strength that I may able to drink it all.

(Diary, 1489)

(Marians of the Immaculate Conception
MARIAN HELPERS
Stockbridge, MA 01263
1-800-462-7426 U.S.A. 1-800-344-2836)

HEAVENLY FATHER

I call on You right now in a special way.
It is through Your power that I was created.

Every breath I take, every morning I wake, and every moment of every hour, I live under Your power.

Father. I ask You now to touch me with that same power. For if You created me from nothing You can certainly recreate me. Fill me with the healing power of Your spirit. Cast out anything that should not be in me. Mend what is broken. Root out any unproductive cells. Open any blocked arteries or veins and rebuild any damaged areas. Remove all inflammation and cleanse any infection.

Let the warmth of Your healing love pass through my body to make new any unhealthy areas so that my body will function the way You created it to function.

And Father, restore me to full health in mind and body so that I may serve You the rest of my life

I ask this through Christ Our Lord. Amen.

(Author Unknown)

THE MIRACLE PRAYER

Lord Jesus, I come before You, just as I am. I am sorry for my sins, I repent of my sins, please forgive me, in Your name. I forgive all others for what they have done against me. I renounce Satan, the evil spirits and all their works. I give You my entire self, Lord Jesus, now and forever. I invite You into my life Jesus, I accept You as my Lord, God

4

SPOUSE, FAMILIES AND FRIENDS OF CANCER SURVIVORS

One of the major concerns of cancer survivors is the difference in the relationship with the most important people in their lives. In many cases they start treating the survivor as a fragile object, one that will break if presented with real life situations. It seems that they are always preparing for the worst, such as the end of life, as if death is near and everyone wants to make you comfortable and offer you various cancer patient stories. The stories often have no real connection to the illness of the survivor.

A spouse is also an important part of the healing process of the survivor. The most important thing the survivor needs is the love, support and encouragement in an environment that has not changed because of this illness. There is a great need to keep things the way they were before the diagnoses of cancer entered the family unit.

The survivor needs the romance, the cuddling, the compliments and the touching. The need for sexuality is even more important now then before, because the survivor wants to be desired by their spouse. Many spouses do not know what to say to the survivor about the disease or how to express their feelings as related to the fear of losing them. Therefore, they go into denial and withdrew from the relationship by becoming silent or even getting involved with someone else, which is often the death of the relationship. Unfortunately, this occurs at a crucial time in the life of a couple when their love should be strongest; this could serve as an opportunity to model love, strength, companionship and real commitment.

The cancer survivor does not want their spouse to become a different person. The only requirement is that they do not allow the fear and feelings of insecurity destroy the relationship that is an important element in the survivor's healing process.

Please do not dismiss the idea of seeking family/marriage counseling, to process the changes within the relationship. The decision may be the most important step in the survivor's recovery. There are many issues involved with the stain of any terminal disease placed on a marriage. There will be temporary changes in the survivor's behavior and the amount of physical activity they will be capable of doing in the early stages of the cancer treatment. This is a time when the spouse's patience, affection and understanding are crucial. There is no need to be concerned about knowing the "RIGHT THING" to say. The key is just to be there, a loving touch on the face or a gentle embrace gives a strong message, even more than any word. The conservation does not necessarily need to always be focused on the survivor's illness. The person's interest in other issues and events has not changed just because of this disease. The survivor is the same person you knew and enjoyed before the cancer diagnoses. Try to focus on the qualities that are the same such as the heart, the mind and the soul.

There are some spouses who act as though they are embarrassed to be seen in public with their mates, particularly when their appearance has changed due to the cancer treatment. Seldom will the spouse verbalize the fact that they are concerned about this trivial form of thinking, nevertheless, their action speaks louder than words. The focus of the matter must be who the most important person here is. Is it Mr. & Mrs. Public, or is it the person that has shared with you the best years of their lives?

The spouse that is an example of true love and devotion in a marriage will ignore the comments of others and provide the needed elements for their mate to successfully heal and become the person they were prior to this illness. The fact is that today it may be your spouse in need of your support, love and patience. But tomorrow it may be you in need of the same treatment from them or someone else. There is a great deal of truth in the cliché that says, "What goes around comes around." In other words, always treat others the way you want to be treated, because, what you give out, always comes back to you in various forms.

The following are suggestions that maybe helpful:

1. Continue to be yourself: a loving friend. Do not try to provide the right answer or a cancer cure.

2. Add humor to the conservations you have with the survivor.

3. Sit near your spouse at home, your presence is most comforting.

4. Listen with interest when your spouse discusses inner feelings, fears and concerns. This will keep both of your spirits up.

5. Encourage your spouse to keep researching new and improved traditional and alternative treatments to counteract this disease.

The marriage vows require a lifetime of commitment. It is so unfortunate that when one of you is attacked with an illness such as cancer that commitment is tested. The positive side of this is that this is an opportunity to learn of your true selves and what you are really made of. The real test is whether you are the person that you would want our spouse to be if the shoe was on the other foot.

The other side of this story is the survivor's attitude, behavior and perception of the impact of cancer on their lives. If the attitude is grounded in strong faith and the belief that they have the power to conquer this disease and continue with their lives, the impact will not be as great. The major problem with many cancer survivors is that they think they are really ill and often use that as an excuse not to be productive and lead full lives. The lives of cancer survivors are not perfect and neither are the lives of people who were never diagnosed with any illness.

Consequently, cancer is only one of those things in our path and the method that each of us selects to use in overcoming those determines the quality of our lives and the future of our relationship with loved ones. The diagnosis of cancer is an opportunity to discover our real strengths and to learn about our unique qualities of spirit. However, the most meaningful lesson is learned when we realize that life is a journey and there will be many turns, road blocks and slopes in our path. Thus, never allow this illness to ruin your opportunity to live the full life God blessed you with at birth.

The best way to cope with any illness is to think positive and believe in the power of God's healing. If you always focus on the negative aspects of cancer, you will end your life years before your death. Never think "What if...." because the end of that phrase is too often on a negative note. The most important thing to remember is that God has given you this day and it is up to you to make the best of it. No one but you has the ability to do this for you, but you.

To the children of cancer survivors, please make every minute you spend with the person you love count as the best possible time you have ever experienced. This will prevent future regrets. The survivor wants you to focus on positive, happy and productive issues. For many reasons negativism is bad for anyone's health and, particularly for cancer survivors, it is a true killer. To adult children of cancer survivors: please do not expect your parents to serve as the sounding board for your problems, hardship or disappointments. The greatest accomplishment of any parent is to know that their children have developed effective strong self-sufficient skills.

The type of essential coping skills that will be a lifeline for the future are: self love, self respect and strong faith in God. When parents recognize that their children have attained these life skills then they can focus on themselves with the comfort of knowing their children will be fine with or without them.

Thus, the cancer survivors are the same people they were prior to being diagnosed. Their needs, thoughts and feelings have not changed, there is only an additional element they are forced to deal with on a daily bases. That is how one keeps winning the fight against this disease. The greatest support family can provide is to take care of themselves by handling their own problems and offering love, kindness and respect to the survivor.

5

MY BREAST CANCER STORY

My name is Glendolyn Duhon Jeanlouis. This is my six-month experience with breast cancer.

Christmas Break was over and the fall semester had just begun. Mrs. Katherine Roede, my curriculum assistant principal, and I were just talking. She asked me if I had my well-woman exam. I told her no because I had been working so diligently on completing my doctoral degree. She picked up the phone and adamantly said, "Call now." That phone call was the beginning of the rest of my life.

January 15, 2004, was Mary Alice Duplechain's, my grandmother's, 94th birthday. I spent the morning at my doctor's office having the first part of the exam and the afternoon was spent at the nursing home at a birthday party for my grandmother. Even though she passed away on October 1, 2004, her love and her spirit will live on forever. After about a week, I hadn't heard anything from my doctor. The following Saturday, I was cleaning off the table and I saw a letter from my doctor's office. I opened it, assuming it was a letter stating that everything was okay. It stated that I needed to call the office immediately, and schedule a mammogram. That Monday morning, I called my doctor, and my mammogram was scheduled for Thursday, February 5, 2004. I had a conversation with my husband, telling him that if they found anything, I wanted to act on it immediately. I had a feeling that something was wrong.

I had the mammogram at River Oaks Imaging that Thursday. It was painful and sort of weird. As the technician was performing the ultrasound, she kept on saying, "I don't see anything." Let me interject at this point that I NEVER felt any pain in my breast. I went home that afternoon and waited to pick up my children from school. About 3:30, the radiologist called, identified himself, and asked me to sit down. He told me that a malignant lump was found in my left breast. I told him that he wasn't a pathologist, and couldn't make a statement like that. He said he knew what he saw, knew how serious it was, and thought I needed to act on it immediately. I said fine, I need to talk to my doctor. She said very softly, "Glendolyn, I am on the line." I told them that if this was as serious as they said, I wanted to see a specialist tomorrow, Friday. My doctor told me to give her twenty minutes, and she would find one for me. While waiting for her call, I called my assistant principal, told her the story, and informed her that I would probably be absent from work the next day. My husband called and said that he would pick up the boys and would see me later. Meanwhile, my doctor's secretary called and set up an appointment with Dr. Henry Glass. She laughed and warned me that he didn't have a good bedside manner. He ended up being a kind gentleman.

I took a deep breath and called my mother. At this time, my mother, who lives in New Orleans, was an eleven-year breast cancer survivor. She was in a meeting, and she said she would call me right back. I told her it was important. About ten minutes later, she called me back. I told her to sit down, and told her the story. I remember her saying, "Whaaat!" She asked if I wanted her to fly down that night and go with me to my doctor's appointment on Friday. I told her that Wendell (my husband) was going with me, and I would keep her informed. She told me later that when we hung up, she told the participants that the meeting was over, and she immediately went home. We talked several times that night. She and my husband believed that since I wasn't hurting, and had no symptoms, that the radiologist was wrong. Both were angry that he had called to worry me about nothing. I called my sisters, Alice and my twin, Gwendolyn. I don't recall their initial reactions. Gwen was a little upset with me because she had had rotator cup surgery in December, and she said that she might not be able to come. Alice was just as concerned, yet neither let on how worried they were. My brother called and said that he would pray for me.

On Friday morning, my husband and I went to see Dr. Glass. Before we met with him, we met with his assistant, Jan. She asked us a million questions, including how soon she should schedule the biopsy. I asked her if there was any way possible that the diagnosis could be wrong. She informed me that he had been a surgeon for 47 years, and he was an expert in the field. I went into the examining room and waited for Dr. Glass. He walked in, and threw the X-ray on the table. He was mumbling to himself, "I know what I know." I have my hand stretched out. I called out his name; he turned around, shook my hand, and went back to mumbling to himself. He then opened a book, and showed me what a malignant lump looked like. Then he placed the X-ray on the lighted screen, and showed me the lump. It looked just like the picture. It resembled a small spider with tentacles. His next question was when I wanted to have the biopsy. He said they would perform the biopsy first, and send it to the pathology lab. If it was malignant, they would perform the mastectomy immediately. I asked if he could do the procedure on the following Monday. He said he needed insurance approval first, and his surgery days were on Tuesdays and Thursdays. So, we set the surgery date for Thursday, February 12, 2004.

I was supposed to fly to Cincinnati that Saturday to meet with my department head to discuss some concerns he had with my dissertation. My mother told me to reschedule, yet I said the reservations were made, and I was going. When I arrived in Cincinnati, it was snowing. It was so beautiful. While waiting for my taxi, I simply stood outside, and allowed the snow to fall upon me. The two days were hectic, and I tried to put the upcoming surgery in the back of my mind. I left that meeting, thinking that I was just going to have to wait until my department head decided to approve my dissertation. It was out of my hands.

I went to school on Monday with so many things to complete. Benchmark tests results, and six weeks' grades were due. Everyone was asking me questions, and giving their advice. Get a second opinion they would say. Some didn't like Dr. Glass. My principal had placed a substitute, Mr. Ross, in my room. He was a sweet, kind, young man. I would work on grades and results, and he would work with the students. I thought that was so sweet of my principal. On Monday afternoon, I emailed my co-workers. I asked them to come to my room and pray with me for my upcoming surgery. There were at least 20 people in my classroom. We held hands in a circle, and just prayed and prayed. You could just feel the power of healing and love in that room. Afterwards, we all hugged, and they left. Many teachers who didn't come emailed me and said that I would be in their thoughts. My family, mother and sisters, were continuing to tell me that this was nothing, and I had nothing to worry about. I would call Jan every morning, and talk to her. She would assure me that I wasn't crazy, and my family would come around. On Tuesday, I called my cousin, Juliet Guillory who was living in Dallas. I told her I needed to talk. I did not know that she wasn't working, and she offered to come and stay with me for the week. She is no longer my cousin, she is now my sister. I told her I needed her to believe with me.

Juliet and my mother arrived Wednesday afternoon, and we began packing for my hospital stay. The doctor told me that if the tumor was benign, the surgery would be same-day surgery. With my mother's disapproval, I packed my suitcase, and took one of my porcelain dolls. I wanted to have something beautiful to look at after surgery. My twin sister met us at the hospital. She and my older sister live in Lake Charles, Louisiana. I told my principal that my husband would call them and let them know whether or not I had breast cancer. I was told later that my older sister came in that afternoon. My mother, Juliet, my twin sister and I recited a rosary before I was wheeled into surgery. I gave my sons the option of coming to the hospital or going to school. Charles chose to come to the hospital; Jordan chose to go to school.

When I came out of surgery, I remember a nurse standing near my bed holding my hand, saying that she was sorry and my left breast was removed. There was a nurse at the foot of my bed with pain medication, Demerol. I was more concerned with pain relief than with the loss of my breast. When I returned to my room, my husband was sitting at the side of my bed. He is a man of very few words. He said, "I'm sorry, I love you, and you are the strongest person I know." Then I didn't see him for a while. My older sister kept staring at me. I later discovered that she was looking at me to see if I was angry over what had just happened. I wasn't though. When the discussion of who was spending the night came up, my husband left the room. My mother spent the night. She had me walking around the room. She had me go to the restroom. The nurse was perturbed with her, yet that didn't stop my mother. In the middle of the night, my blood vessel popped, and they had to take out the IV. I don't have good veins. The nurses said they would wait until morning to put another IV line in if needed. Every time someone would come into my hospital room, they would comment on how beautiful my porcelain doll was. My mother bought me another one to add to my collection.

The next morning, I had to have tests run to determine if the surgeon had gotten all of the tumor and the infected lymph nodes. After the tests, the nurses came and said that I was going home. My mother was so upset. She thought that I wasn't ready to go home. The patient coordinator came to my room, and told me that I had done everything they needed done; I had no fever, and was able to go home. That weekend cousins, my assistant principal, friends, and co-workers came to visit. The phone never stopped ringing.

I was fortunate enough to get cancer insurance through my school district. I thought that I was going to get ahead of the game, and send my records in ahead of time. It still took six weeks for the first check to come. I would call the customer service number daily. I complained to the district insurance representative. Waiting was the worst part of all. Thank God for my mother. She helped my family get through the month that I didn't get paid. She sent vitamins such as shark cartilage, flaxseed oil, selenium, anti-oxidants, glucosamine, grape seed oil, cranberry, and Chinese herbal tea.

Juliet cared for me the first week. She had to change my drains twice a day. I was taking medicine for pain, so I was sleeping often. She would come into the room and watch me sleep. She would fix strawberries and bananas for me for breakfast. I had to ride with her to pick up the boys from school. She was also looking for a job. I told her that because of what she was doing for me, God would get her the perfect job for her. She was offered a job by the end of that week. My husband tried to help. He decided the best way for him to help me was to take care of the boys. I remember how my sons would come into my room nightly and ask me if I was all right. My youngest son would lie at the foot of my bed just to be near me.

I started a journal about this time, because of my mother's urging. We took a lot of pictures at this time as well. Keeping busy seemed to lift my spirits.

Juliet left on Saturday, February 22, 2004. Gwen took over the shift for the weekend. Wendell took the boys to his mother's house in Jeanerette, Louisiana. Gwen and Grace met Juliet and I at the clothing store. She didn't recognize me. She was looking for a sickly looking woman. I had sunglasses on and was happy. Gwen and I spoke of healing and love for each other. My friend Chelensky met us at the house. She was such a jewel. She cleaned and cleaned, and fussed at Wendell for not cleaning. She is a true friend.

I sat in front of the television set watching Sunday mass. I thanked God for keeping me alive and for all of my family and friends. My mother prepared pill packets and my sister folded clothes. We purchased curtains to change the look of my living room. I was dealing with nausea then, and was determined to win. After swallowing my pill pack, I caught the chills. Then I had to put on socks, a robe, and a bed spread. Mama prepared an okra gumbo, and was preparing containers of gumbo for me to eat daily. Gwen gave me beautiful gifts.

I wasn't sleeping for very long then, yet when I did, I felt rested. Fighting cancer made me appreciate what things were important like watching my sons prepare for school, and family time together. My mother would fuss because she thought I wasn't resting enough.

My birthday came on February 24, 2004. It started out with a bang. My boys sang. My husband prepared breakfast. My mother prepared my favorite dish, okra gumbo. My oldest sister and my niece sang. My menstrual cycle started. I haven't had another cycle to this day. The doctor said that the chemotherapy might thrust me into menopause. I believe it has.

My team sent me a beautiful card. I received a call from Dr. Green, the vice president of the university from which I received my Ph.D., telling me not to worry, that he would call my department head, Dr. Preston.

February 26 proved to be a day filled with ups and downs. I was worried about the money, yet I continued to believe that God would see me through. He did! I started that day with reading Psalms. Juliet called me from Oakland. Miss Hattie, from cancer recovery, came by and gave me a pillow and some cancer material. She asked me to volunteer to talk to other cancer survivors. I thought doing this would help me to heal. Our insurance agent, Abner Brown, came by, took pictures of the work done on the house, and told me of his experience with prostate cancer. Later that afternoon, Mrs. Figaro, my other assistant principal, and Mrs. Jordan, our school secretary, came by and brought a beautiful plant. Chelensky called to check on me.

The next day started at 3:30 a.m. with me trying to make sure that my son, Jordan didn't have fever. Mission accomplished, it broke. I took a cool shower, and washed my hair. Joann, my beautician and close friend, came and styled my hair. I looked beautiful! I fasted and prayed. I was waiting for fish for lunch.

The next day, Sunday, was spent alone. I was waiting for Vicky, a teacher on my team at school, to bring the dinner that my team purchased for me. Melanie, my cousin, wanted to go furniture shopping. Yet, because I was feeling ill, I declined, and felt guilty about it.

I deemed the week of March to be "Hell Week." I understood what the meaning of insurance red tape meant, and I had run-ins with the customer service people of the Internal Revenue Service. I stupidly and naively thought that insurance companies would pay quickly. NOT! I was trying to handle things myself. I messed that up as well. It was funny how I thought I could take responsibility for myself when problems arose. I still needed my mother's help. Yet perhaps that was a blessing as well.

Father Alphonses, my church priest, would come and pray with me every Monday. I continued to swallow my tea, and my vitamins. Friends continued to come by to give moral support, and love. My twin couldn't wait to shave her head. She, my mother, and my older sister continued to call every day.

I began my first visit to M.D. Anderson Hospital on March 15, 2004, which incidentally was the first day of Spring Break. Who else would have been there with me except for Gwendolyn? On the way to the hospital, I was ready to have a good cry. Due to the fact that Gwen was lost, she told me not now. So by the time we found our way, the moment had passed and we laughed about it. Registration was a breeze. The people were so nice. Then they sent us to Dr. Pusvtai's office. He told me the name of my cancer: insitu ductal carcinoma. I couldn't have enjoyed it or gotten through it without Gwen. As Dr. Pusvtai was telling me the course of treatment that he prepared which included 3 months of regular chemotherapy, and three months of "triple chemo," which is a triple dose of the regular chemotherapy treatment. He told me that most people take two weeks to decide what they will do. I asked if the treatment could start that day. He laughed, and said the treatment would start the following Friday. That afternoon we had to attend CVC class. This class shows cancer patients how to care for the line from which the patient receives chemotherapy. I believe it was at this point that it all came tumbling down. I began to fidget; the film seemed scary, and I had to leave the room. The nurse understood and was very patient. I was trying to be strong and do everything on that day. I just kept on saying "I can do all things through Christ that strengthens me."

Well, on I went. Normally when I jump into something I do it with both feet. Whatever was going to happen, I knew God would be at my side. Watching the CVC film brought reality to life. Knowing what was going to happen, then seeing and hearing it was two different things. I cried. I just continued believing that I would get through it.

On Wednesday of that week, I had to go to the hospital alone. I had tests to get done. Jesus was with me, along with all of those other patients with a predicament similar to mine. I left my cell phone in the car. The valet attendant walked to the parking garage to retrieve it for me. Mama allowed me to talk to her, telling her how I felt without holding anything back. Wendell wouldn't talk a lot then. I thought it was because I snapped at him.

My first day of chemotherapy started out great. It was 5:30 a.m. and we were ready to go. I saw my grandmother, and she promised to pray for me.

The afternoon chemotherapy session went superb. I was so relaxed. I kept feeling my angels all around me. I had a short episode of shortness of breath. The nurse came and added Benadryl. Things began to slow down. I started taking slow, deep breaths, and the episode went away. The cafeteria staff brought in lunch, which made the chemotherapy experience better. Gwen made the experience bearable and not so scary.

March 20, 2004 was my eleventh wedding anniversary and twenty-four hours after chemotherapy. It began at 5:00 a.m. Wendell and I talked quietly and nicely together. Then the house woke up and I started getting ready for the hospital. Twenty-four hours after the CVC line is inserted, it has to be rechecked and the bandage has to be changed. Jordan was sulking because he had to miss his first baseball game. The doctor had ordered X-rays to see if Jordan had pneumonia, and he had just started taking his antibiotics. I began fussing because Wendell was insisting that Jordan would be all right. I then began feeling guilty for stopping him from going to the game. When we arrived at the hospital, and told the nurse about our argument, she told Wendell that Jordan could have passed out and died if he had gone to that game. Wendell just needed to hear it from a professional. I spent the rest of the day resting. Mama fixed an awesome soup.

The next day, Sunday, I awoke early and dressed. Then I woke up my mother. It is always sad to see her go. She bought so many things to improve the quality of life for me. After she left, I attended Mass and it was so uplifting.

My older sister was dating a very, kind young man named Cedric at that time. His first visit to my house was nurturing and spiritual. Cedric's sister had died two years ago from breast cancer. He told me that listening to Alice talk about me and my condition reminded him of the story of the mulberry tree from the Bible. In his Bible, it spoke about having faith the size of a mustard seed, and the strength of a mulberry tree. A mulberry tree can grow anywhere. You can uproot it, replant it and it will survive. When I first heard him refer to me as a mulberry tree, I was offended. But I was spiritually moved after hearing the whole story.

I wanted to capture moments during my cancer journey. I bought a camera to capture these moments. After six weeks of being home recovering, the day came for me to report back to work. I was ready. I was tired of being in the house, and was ready to make some money. That day was exhilarating and exhausting. I took that day one hour at a time. Everyone was so glad to see me and had mixed emotions about my hair. I had been slowly cutting it shorter, preparing myself for when it would fall out. I turned in lesson plans. Mrs. Earls, the sixth grade assistant principal, came and offered me respite when I became tired. I just sort of felt my way the entire day. Some classes completed more work than others did.

That afternoon I had an appointment with Dr. Glass. He said my stitches looked well, there was no more fluid, and he would see me in six months.

On Tuesday, I received flowers from the counselors, more hugs from my co-workers, words of encouragement, and good work from my students. I brought my pictures to be mounted, and brought Jordan to church for first communion practice. I lay down about 9:30, exhausted and a little sore, and went to sleep. The counselors were constantly asking me if I needed any help. As the week progressed, I gained more energy, and accomplished more. I was so thrilled to complete my first week.

My second chemotherapy treatment was great. Mrs. Holcombe, my friend, came with me. My blood pressure didn't go up. I came home and took a nap.

The last day in March is a happy day in my family. It is my youngest son's birthday. This year it was even more special, because my doctoral diploma arrived in the mail. Seven years of graduate school were finally over. I didn't allow my illness to stop my dream.

Dr. Postal gave me great news during my April visit. He said that microscopically they could not find any more traces of cancer in my body. I began crying. I called my mother from the doctor's office, and she began crying. I credit prayer, taking the vitamins, drinking the tea, and my will to continue on no matter what.

On Easter Sunday, my worst fears came true. I had had one month of chemotherapy without any hair loss. I was lying on my mother's hotel room bed. When I got up to leave, there was lots of hair on the pillow. My son Charles said, "Mom, look!!!" I really was sad to begin to lose my hair. But, like everything I had been through, I went to Wal-Mart the next day and told the lady in the salon to shave it. When she was about finished, I told Charles to go and pick up a can of starch. I told him that because I didn't have a scarf, I wouldn't be able to go into the store. The beautician quickly told me I was beautiful and didn't need a scarf. She continued to say that I had nothing to be ashamed of, and because I was still alive, I was a winner. Well, that was all that it took. I have been stepping out ever since. I went home that evening, called Gwen, and told her the story. She immediately informed me that she had shaved her head the day before, and what took me so long.

Well, the next day I was back to school. I wore a hat to cover my shaved head. My student, Anna, told me to take my hat off because they loved me just the way I was, hair or no hair. My bald head shocked some of my co-workers. Some offered to buy me a wig. I refused. I began to enjoy my own head, and haven't worn a wig since that day.

Mother's Day, 2004, was an awesome day. It ended up being the last Mother's Day that we spent with my grandmother. Mama, Mom Alice, and I spent the afternoon laughing and laughing. Easter dinner was at my house, and it was delicious. Alice and I went out and drank margaritas. I didn't know when I had more fun. Alice bought me the most beautiful Circle of Angel's candle. Mama gave me two watches. She loved the potpourri pot and scent and the knitted picture that I had given her. It was a family day full of love; a glorious, super blessed day.

I would continue to go to chemotherapy every Saturday, and see my doctor once a month until June. He would tell me that I needed to stop working, or start wearing a mask if I continued to work. I couldn't quit for financial reasons, and I couldn't put on a mask. I thought it would make me look sicker than I actually was. I had nausea the evening after chemotherapy, and the Sunday as well. I swallowed my nausea medicine religiously, and slept most of the weekend. I would be really tired Monday and Tuesday, yet by Wednesday I was full of energy again. Those vitamins and the tea really strengthened me and my immune system.

The school year ended. Our scores were lower than they had ever been since I had been at Eckert. Yet, I had the highest math scores in the school. I was so blessed.

Summer began, and I was determined to teach summer school. Summer school lasted only twenty days. My doctor had warned me that the triple chemotherapy treatments would cause me to be sicker, and would totally exhaust me. My family came through for me. My mother kept my sons the first two weeks of summer. My sister kept Jordan the last two weeks of summer school. I did get sick. I had to change the CVC line twice. Yet, I continued to persevere, and this was the best summer school session that I had worked. I was able to team teach with the other math teacher. During the summer, when I was feeling my lowest, my mother would tell me to write or type what I was feeling.

August 16, 2004, was the third day of school in my district, and where was I? I was at home, weak, nauseous, and wishing not to be sick. I had the CVC line taken off for two weeks. Apparently, I didn't enjoy it enough. My right shoulder area was sore; I was going to the bathroom constantly, and I wanted a new life free of chemotherapy. I had lost a little weight; that's gone. I am now up to 269 pounds, which is not a very sexy weight. I want to stay home and get better slowly, like I did this summer when I undertook the second chemo treatment. I didn't want to go to school the next day looking for pity. I wanted to be strong, beautiful, and pain free. There was a fat chance of that happening.

In the beginning of my "triple chemo sessions," I was strong; I could talk about my illness, and thought that I could help people. My brother, Patrick, came with me to my last chemotherapy session. We talked and laughed about problems we were having in our own families. He was so happy to see me finish my chemo. He had to leave early, but we hugged before he left. I was sitting there waiting for my ride, and I began talking to a lady who was going through chemo treatment with her mother. The lady was happy for me that I was finished.

6

RECOMMENDATION FOR THE NEW LIFE OF CANCER SURVIVORS

The first step in the new life of a cancer survivor is to believe deep in your heart that you are not a victim. This is a serious illness that unfortunately you have incurred, as have over a million other people across the nation. This diagnosis is not because of something you did or did not do. This cancer is not a form of punishment from God because you were either a bad or a good person or of a certain size, color or cultural group. Cancer is an illness you have and you must believe that you will live a beautiful, long and healthy life in the aftermath of this illness, as many others have.

The mind, the way you perceive the cancer experience or think about yourself as a cancer survivor often determines your success in the healing process. There will be days when you may require extra effort to do the simple tasks which used to be so easy for you to perform without thinking. Please do not allow that to slow you down or cause you to quit trying new things and developing your new skills and things you enjoy. The process may be a little difficult in the beginning, but every time you push yourself the task becomes easier. Always view yourself as the same person you were before the cancer; nothing has changed. You are only healthier now because your body has been tested for every possible disease.

The key to a successful recovery is to share your story with other people who are interested. I have not met one person since I had cancer who doesn't know at least one family member or friend who is suffering or has suffered with cancer. For that reason, many people are interested in learning how you found the strength to bounce back from this illness stronger and more eager to receive life's gifts than ever. When telling your story, focus on the positive and describe the hard times as challenges you have conquered and learned great life lessons from.

The level of confidence you express will lift the spirit of others who are struggling with a new diagnosis of this thing called cancer.

The major focus of a cancer survivor should be on developing new skills to enjoy life at its highest level, with a new insight and determination to be happy and healthy. The flowers, cool air and different sweet smells in a garden of vegetables or fruit trees. The small pleasures of life are so important that we often take them for granted. They may have a new meaning when focusing on capitalizing on all of God's Gifts to us in this life. Make a special effort to thank God for the little blessings, such as a warm smile from a child or a stranger, or someone holding the door for you. Please allow yourself to enjoy helping others in small ways. For example, when someone is walking your way, smile and greet them even when they do not respond. It feels good to be the strong, positive person with the courage to see God in all human beings. Please stop to smell the roses and see God's smile in the mean, angry and evil faces. Those people who are "poor in spirit" need your help to struggle through the day. You have a special Gift from God in that you have experienced cancer in your body and now you are healed. Now you are a model, one who has the strength to comfort others who may be weak due to a lack of understanding that cancer is not always the killer as viewed by many. Please repeat five times: "God has healed my body so that I may live and enjoy life to its fullest." This prayer will help you to relax, and you will sense a level of peace that will help you to deal with many of cancer's complications.

One of the most dangerous emotions for a cancer survivor is anger. Anger blocks the flow of health, healing and peace of mind. This may sound strange or even crazy, but think about how you feel when you are really angry. Your muscles tighten up, your heart beats faster, and hate and rage dominate your thinking. This may cause the cells in your body to function in an unnatural manner that may lead to serious illness. The most important thing is to decide that you will not allow anyone or anything to drive you to anger. There are many situations in life that may generate feelings of anger, but when you are determined to block that negative emotion from hurting you, you are in control. There are many effective ways to be in control of your emotions. Try the following strategies:

A. Ask yourself this question: "Is this a real issue or am I displacing aggression from something else in my life?"

B. Consider the value of getting angry or finding an effective solution to the real problem. Will your anger change this situation in a positive way?

C. Write five reasons why getting angry may effect your day in a negative way.

1. Changing your demeanor, realizing that your attitude determines your emotional stability whether it is negative or positive.

2. Consider the source of the behavior of the person or people that is creating the negativity in your life.

3. The old ways you learned as a child still works: count to 10 and take 5 deep breaths.

4. Call the name of Jesus 5 times in your heart and at the end of that smile and know that He is comforting you, so try to relax.

5. Visualize yourself as a butterfly and you are flying above and beyond the present situation.

Try these other visualizations:

A. Close your eyes and view yourself sitting near the river and the water is washing all the mean or bad things away.

B. Sing a beautiful song of love and happiness in your heart, without uttering a word.

C. Focus on the first smile or first step of a baby and how that makes parents feel.

D. View yourself helping an elderly person and the appreciation that glows in their eyes and on their faces.

E. Contact the person that offended you and discuss the problem, explaining your understanding of the problem, how you feel about it and offer a solution to enhance forward movement with a stronger relationship.

F. The best strategy of all is to surround yourself with positive, loving and kind people who have strong people skills, individuals who really believe in the power of God and recognize that He walks with us through our daily problems, and carries us through our daily struggle.

Always have plans for a fun event, something to look forward to for the next day or week or month. Acknowledge all Holidays, and whenever possible, go all the way with decorations. Invite relatives and friends who you enjoy being around. Daily, find things to laugh about and make others laugh. One of the best places to visit and laugh and make others laugh is the park or playground where children are playing.

On a daily basis, work on your appearance. When you look great, it is easy to feel great. Sometimes wearing an outfit you haven't worn lately makes you feel like a brand new person and very special. Always focus on wearing bright colors and cheery clothes that are very comfortable. Often the clothes you wear may be the essential tool to lift up your spirits. Please remember the most important accessory is a smile!

Develop an action plan that includes daily, weekly, monthly and yearly activities to organize, attend or participate. Join various groups in church, community or local schools. This will help you to reach out, meet new people and contribute to improving the quality of life of others. Make at least one phone call daily to a person who is really excited to talk with you about you. This may be a relative, a friend or an elderly person who loves you just for who you are today.

Fight the temptation to feel fearful of the future. Fear breeds hopelessness, despair and misery. When the thought of death or dying enters your mind, think of it as a new beginning. This is the time to focus on the gift of life as always renewing itself and death as a form of renewal in the spiritual sense. Cancer is a disease, not an automatic killer. There are people who have survived cancer for over fifty (50) years. The key element in successful healing is the ability to control the fear by living life to its fullest. Please keep away from those who are eager to tell you the names of those who have died of cancer. There are those who mention people who've recently died of cancer whenever they encounter cancer survivors. Actually, some of them are only ignorant and do not mean to hurt you; they are not aware of the impact of their words. Therefore, you need to tell them in very positive terms that you do not need to be reminded that people die of cancer, as some do of other illnesses. Your real friends will be delighted for your honesty and the others may have had the wrong intentions, they may not be real friends. Develop new, different and exciting skills. Take lessons in areas you felt you did not have time or energy to do before. Enroll in a ballroom dancing class or something in the arts. This is your time to re-invent yourself into that beautiful, loving, courageous and positive person God meant you to be in this world.

The book is designed to help people accept and understand that a diagnosis of cancer is not a death sentence. Often you have the ability to determine the results. It is a signal to help recognize the good, the beauty, and the value of living a healthy, full-filled life each day if you decide what is experienced and viewed as the positive value of each occurrence. The greatest reward in life is to give of our knowledge of conquering cancer to others. The key to this is to recognize the small daily blessings and to view each one as a source of joy. The perception of the reason why one has incurred cancer has control over anything that happens to that person. If one believes that the cancer was the result of being mean or a bad person or committed some kind of sin, that negative thinking will destroy the positive efforts to heal the body. The news of having a cancerous tumor in my body required me to take action. I needed to do something. There were several different approaches I could choose to take, such as:

1. Sit around feeling sorry for myself, asking "why me?"

2. Move into denial and work on protecting the secret, wishing it would go away.

3. Trust in God, pray for guidance, while I take charge of my health through traditional, alternative cancer treatments.

4. Research everything written about cancer, read and reread and discuss it with other cancer survivors, family and friends.

5. Explore new treatments and ask many questions of professionals. You will be surprised at the number of people you know who have had cancer and are keeping the secret.

6. Start daily exercise, even if it is only for five (5) minutes in the beginning.

7. Go to the library to check out a yoga exercise tape.

8. Check the web sites for material on positive visual imaging to help the mind visualize and see a fully healthy body functioning at the highest level of a full life.

9. Check the web to get involved with daily discussions with positive thinking cancer survivors who are eager to share the path they took in their journey to winning the cancer battle.

10. Recognize your gift of self-actualization and decide how to use your gift to enhance the quality of life of another person who may be struggling with the initial news of the diagnosis of cancer.

The major thrust of the information in this book is to soften the blow of the diagnosis of cancer and to help everyone to realize that cancer does not have to be a tragedy; it may be converted into your gift of self-actualization. It depends on the perception you develop based on your attitude.

978-0-595-43090-1
0-595-43090-2